The Ultimate Keto Diet for Beginners

Keto that Fits Your Lifestyle

By

Vonnie Lynn

Contents

The Ultimate Keto Diet for Beginners

Keto That Fits Your Lifestyle

Chapter 5: The Recipes

Lunch Recipes

Dinner Recipes

Dessert Recipes

About the Author:

Book Description

Do you find yourself carrying a few extra pounds? Is there a special event coming up for which you would like to slim down and look your best? A wedding? A reunion? Is obesity affecting your health, hurting your joints, or throwing your blood sugar out of balance? The Keto Diet is a safe and proven way to lose not only pounds, but also excess body fat quickly.

This book contains proven strategies and information to help you lose weight in a short period of time.-, plus some surprising ways Keto is being used to treat certain medical conditions.

Nothing in this book should be considered to be medical advice, and I highly recommend consulting your physician before beginning any diet or exercise program, especially if you have an underlying health condition.

The Ultimate Keto Diet for Beginners includes delicious, affordable, and simple recipes to keep your Keto diet interesting. In this book, you will learn tips on how to effectively apply the keto diet to your lifestyle, follow a meal plan, and prepare a variety of delicious breakfast dishes, main course meals, snacks and sides, and more.

The Ketogenic diet is tested and proven through the decades to help you lose weight quickly and effectively. Get started now and enjoy the benefits of becoming lean and feeling great.

Introduction

Ketosis diet plans, also known as ketogenic diets, feature foods that are surprisingly low in carbs.

One's body depends upon carbs as its primary energy source. As your body processes carbohydrates, their energy is released and is used to fuel your body. Whenever you limit your consumption of carbs, your system has no "easy" fuel to burn, which makes it look for other sources. To keep your body going, it turns to stored fat.

A diet which causes your body to consume fat for energy will not only help you lose weight; **it will also help you lose fat.** The Keto Diet does just this.

It's a no-brainer!

Some individuals say that ketogenic diet plans are dangerous. They really are _very_ safe; the problem is that some people confuse the words "ketoacidosis" and "ketogenic."

Ketoacidosis is very dangerous and only happens in individuals who have diabetes, once the amount of sugar in their blood goes out of control. Naturally, we do not like to conflate these two words.

Ketosis has been proven to not only assist in your struggle to lose weight, but it also helps ward off illness.

* * * * *

Plenty of research has existed on ketogenic diet plans concerning obesity.

In virtually every study, the individuals on a ketogenic diet plan reported that their appetites appeared to decrease. This reduction happens because ketogenic diets are naturally very high in protein.

Protein plays a crucial role in how soon we start to feel full, that, of course, makes you much less hungry.

Furthermore, scientists have found that people who were eating a low-fat diet regime needed to actively curb their calorie intake. But people consuming a low-carb diet regime got the same results as those in the low-fat group, yet they didn't have to be as diligent in tracking their calorie consumption.

Most reduced-carb diet plans tend to have plenty of saturated fats, which, by reputation, are not healthy for us.

Even with the higher saturated fat consumption, men and women consuming a low carbohydrate diet plan had improved HDL cholesterol and triglyceride levels, as well as less insulin resistance.

* * * *

For children with epilepsy, studies have shown there are benefits to a strong ketogenic diet plan. Due to the lower carbs, these people tend to have a smaller number of seizures.

One study revealed that 38% of children on a ketogenic diet plan had a 50% decrease in the frequency of their seizures, and 7% had more than a 90% reduction. With all these excellent results, you would think that Keto would be a household word, and while nearly everyone has heard of Keto, *few know what it entails.*

On a ketogenic diet you will eat a Low-carbohydrate, high-fat, moderate protein menu. Only 5% or so of your calories will come from carbs, roughly 20-50 grams/day. When you eat this way, your body produces ketones to burn for energy instead of using glucose.

When I say you should consume 20 to 50 grams, I'm referring to net carbs rather than total carbs. Some carbohydrates such as sugar alcohols and fiber don't increase blood glucose levels. Here's heow to figure net carbohydrates:

Look at the nutrition label on a product. You will usually see entries for "Total Carbohydrates," "Dietary Fiber," and "sugars"

Total carbs minus grams of dietary fiber minus grams of sugar alcohol equals net carbs.

So your diet may include Total Carbs higher than 5% of your diet, but your net carbs will still need to stay under the 5% threshold.

A word about MACROS:

"Macros", slang for *macronutrients*, are the nutrients you need for your body to thrive. The three main macros are fat, protein, and carbohydrates, and are usually expressed as percentages of your caloric intake. The typical diet in the U.S. consists of around 35% fat, 15% protein, and 50% carbohydrates. *That's right, **half** of our diet is carbohydrates!*

The macros for a keto diet are 75% fat, 20% protein, and 5% carbs. You can make figuring out your macros as complicated as you wish, or you can keep it simple. There are apps you can use to track your macros, (especially helpful at first while you are learning the diet), after which you can ease into "lazy keto" where you keep a running total in your head as you listen to your body and learn what makes you feel good. You may also use "The Ultimate Keto Diet Workbook" to keep track of your macros and help you along your keto journey.

A few tips to help ensure your success are to keep it simple, plan ahead, and to eat "real" foods.

The more we overthink things, the less likely we are to follow through with them. We're all about fitting keto into our lifestyle, not fitting our life into keto, right? Let's not make this any more complicated than we have to. What the keto diet boils down to is that we curtail the number of carbs we eat. With a little bit of planning we can remove the things that will tempt us from our pantries, make sure that we have foods available that will not sabotage our efforts, and as much as possible avoid processed or pre-packaged foods which often contain hidden sugars.

In the following chapters you will learn some surprising benefits to following a ketogenic diet that extend far beyond weight loss. It is my hope that you will find my book is a helpful guide on your weight loss journey and that you will find it informative and inspiring. At the end of the book you will find some contact information. I would love to hear your success stories!

-Vonnie

Chapter 1: What is a Ketogenic Diet?

The ketogenic diet is a low-carb, high-fat, and high protein diet that burns fat to generate energy for the body. **The maximum limit for carbohydrates is 5% of your total calorie intake**. Figuring this out can be a little tricky, so the rule of thumb is no more than 50g of carbs per day.

Keto is an easy diet to follow for those who love their protein. Eating meats, cheeses, and other high-fat/high-protein (and, therefore, high-taste!) foods is the order of the day. It focuses on drastically cutting carb intake, which then forces the body into the ketosis state.

The Ketosis state is a natural process of the body where the body breaks down food in a slower manner than our body is accustomed to and begins to burn that unsightly fat that we've stored up for a rainy day.

Open your umbrellas!

Benefits of a Keto Diet

Research has shown the ketogenic diet to be a great way to lose weight. That's fine and dandy, but losing weight shouldn't be the only thing you seek with a diet. You should have more energy and better indications of health, such as lower cholesterol. Starting a ketogenic diet *may* improve your health in addition to losing weight. ***Consult your doctor, though, before making any drastic changes to your health regime.***

Here are a few conditions that seem to be helped by a Ketogenic Diet:

Prevention of diabetes:

Diabetes is essentially an impaired function of how your body uses insulin. Studies have shown the ketogenic diet to be able to improve insulin sensitivity.

The higher your insulin sensitivity levels are, the less insulin your body will require to lower blood glucose levels back to normal. Your body doesn't burn fat when insulin levels are high. Therefore, it's important to improve insulin sensitivity levels to help better regulate blood glucose levels.

Lower risk for heart disease:

Heart disease is one of the leading causes of death in the United States. It includes many risk factors such as cholesterol levels, body fat, blood sugar, and blood pressure. The ketogenic diet can help to improve these risk factors, thus lowering the risk of heart disease.

Getting rid of acne:

Another cool side benefit is that this diet can help you get rid of acne if you struggle with breakouts regularly. The ketogenic diet will help to lower insulin levels by eating less processed foods and sugar, which can help prevent acne.

Cancer treatment:

The ketogenic diet is currently being used to treat several different types of cancer, and it can slow tumor growth. Of course, more research is needed for conclusive evidence, but early results are promising.

Increase HDL cholesterol levels:

There are two different kinds of cholesterol HDL (which stands for high-density lipoproteins and LDL which stands for low-density lipoproteins.)

Your HDL is your good cholesterol that you want to increase because it is responsible for carrying cholesterol to the liver, where it can then be excreted or reused.

LDL's, on the other hand, are the bad cholesterol and are responsible for carrying cholesterol away from the liver and into the body. Research shows that one of the best ways to increase your HDL levels is to increase your fat intake. You'll easily be able to achieve that with the standard ketogenic protocol of 75% of your calories coming from fat.

Lower blood pressure:

Lowering your carbohydrate intake has been shown to decrease hypertension. Having higher blood pressure increases your risk of developing diseases such as heart disease and stroke.

Decrease triglyceride levels:

Triglycerides are fat molecules. It might sound counter-intuitive that increasing your fat intake would decrease the number of triglycerides in the blood, but it really does. The reduction occurs because carbs are one of the most significant contributors to increasing triglycerides. Therefore, by decreasing carb intake, you'll reduce the triglycerides in your blood.

More weight loss than a typical diet:

Studies have shown that people who restrict calories on a low-carb diet lose more weight and lose weight faster than individuals restricting calories on a low-fat diet. The main reason for this is because low-carb diets lower insulin levels, which will cause the body to get rid of excess sodium within the first few weeks of starting the diet.

A positive way to lose your appetite:

When you go on most diets and restrict your calories, you start to feel hungry.

If your feelings of hunger begin to get out of control, you're more likely to give up on your diet.

Obviously, if you go back to your old habits, you have no chance of losing weight and improving your health.

Luckily, the Keto diet has been shown to decrease appetite. This is critical because it'll allow you to lower your overall caloric intake without having to worry about getting extra hungry. And eating savory, protein-laden foods are encouraged.

You may miss the sugar initially, but there are good substitutes to use so that you don't feel deprived.

Foods to Avoid:

Processed foods

- Tropical fruit: papaya, banana, pineapple

- Sugar, honey

- Alcoholic drinks: beer, cocktails,

- Refined fats/oils, e.g., grape seed, corn oil, sunflower

<h1 style="text-align:center"><u>Foods to Eat</u>:</h1>

- **Healthy fats**
- Monounsaturated (olive, macadamia, and avocado oil)

-

- Saturated (goose fat, tallow, clarified butter/ghee, coconut oil, duck fat, lard, butter, chicken fat)

- Polyunsaturated omega 3s (seafood and fatty fish)

- Artificial Sweeteners: Stevia, Erythritol, Sucralose, Xylitol

Non-starchy vegetables:

- Kale

- Lettuce

- Bamboo Shoots

- Celery Stalk

- Asparagus

- Cucumber

- Spinach

- Zucchini

- Radishes

- Chives

- Endive

Fruits:

- Watermelon

- Berries

- Avocado

- Mangoes

Nuts and seeds:

- Hemp seeds

- Pine nuts

- Pecans

- Almonds

- Sunflower seeds

- Macadamia nuts

- Walnuts

- Pumpkin seeds

- Hazelnuts

- Sesame seeds

Dairy Products:

- Whole milk yogurt (unsweetened)

- Heavy whipping cream

- Cream cheese

Beverages:

- Water

- Unsweetened coconut milk

- Unsweetened soymilk

- Coffee

- Unsweetened almond milk

- Unsweetened herbal tea

- Unsweetened herbal tea

Proteins/Meats:

- Poultry: Chicken meat, duck meat, and quail meat

- Shellfish: Squid, Clams, scallops, lobster, mussels, crab, and oysters,

- Meat: Goat, Beef, Lamb, and other wild game

- Fish: cod, halibut, tuna, salmon, trout, flounder, mackerel, snapper, and catfish.

- Whole Eggs

- Sausage and bacon

- Pork products

Spices:

- Cayenne Pepper

- Black Pepper

- Cumin

- Rosemary

- Parsley

- Basil

- Thyme

- Sea salt

- Sage

- Oregano

As you can see, there are plenty of tasty foods and snacks that you can eat and still get your body into ketosis. Just be sure to keep your carb count under 50g/day, and you should be in ketosis within 2 days to a couple of weeks.

Chapter 2: Dos and Don'ts of a Ketogenic Diet

If you are not familiar with the keto diet, mistakes can be made to keep you from having good health and the benefits of this diet. To enhance the success with the ketogenic diet, here are some dos and don'ts about following the diet:

Do Exercise when convenient:

If you are the exercising type, you should continue to exercise while on the ketogenic diet. One of the things that makes the Keto diet so popular is that you can successfully lose weight without working out.

There is a misconception, however, that you shouldn't exercise while doing Keto. You may continue (or start) light to moderate exercise while on Keto. However, if you are very active, or a bodybuilder, you should consume more carbs than a person on keto who isn't physically active.

Your body will need the energy those few extra carbs give to get you through the workout without feeling fatigued. A feeling of tiredness is common in the early stages of Keto, as your body adapts to using ketones for fuel rather than glucose. Stay the course! Within a few days your energy level will return. If you feel too lethargic, add a little bit of fruit such as blueberries or raspberries as snacks, just don't overdo it!

Don't worry.

You will blow through those carbs quickly, and get back to burning fat. If you are *extremely* physically active, you may consider the three-day carb-loading cycle described later in the book.

The use of exercise while dieting helps in the restoration of your muscle mass, energy, and keeping fit. You can skip the workouts and still lose weight, but your results will come faster with a little exercise thrown in. If you cannot get into the gym, you can buy a workout DVD or download a workout video to your cell that you can use in your home.

Do Watch your calories:

This is very important to the successful completion of your ketogenic diet challenge. Limit the number of calories that you take in. Too many will not only ruin your results but also store up in your body. You will gain weight instead of losing it. So, watch your calorie intake in order to get the desired result.

The ketogenic diet is a low-carb diet, which means you should lower your carb intake. A specific number of carbs you should have in a diet is not there. Many people follow a diet where they consume 100 to 150 grams of carbs a day. To achieve ketosis, be sure that your carbohydrate intake is low. Most keto dieters manage the state of ketosis by consuming between 20 to 100 grams of carbs a day.

Don't be scared of fats, especially healthy fats like Omega-3s, monounsaturated fats, and saturated fats. Eating fats is encouraged in the ketogenic diet plan; a limit of 60 to 70% fat intake is best. To achieve these levels of fat, you must consume meat and healthy fats, such as olive oil, lard, butter, and coconut or alternatives daily.

If you don't have time to cook, you may turn to fast foods. Don't even think about it.

Fast foods are incredibly unhealthy and can deter you from your keto journey. Fast foods contain too many harmful chemicals and preservatives, and some fast foods use processed cheese and meats that contain hidden sugars.

Protein is an essential nutrient that your body needs. It can soothe your appetite and burn fat more than any other nutrient. Generally, protein is said to be very useful for weight loss, increased muscle mass, and improved body composition.

By reducing carbohydrate consumption, your insulin levels fall, which in turn reduces the sodium stored in your body. If you experience sodium deficiency, you might have symptoms of exhaustion, headaches, constipation, etc. To relieve this problem, increase your sodium intake on a keto diet. Add a teaspoon of salt to daily meals or drink a glass of water with a ¼ teaspoon of salt mixed with it.

It is common for us to seek immediate gratification. When you start a diet, you may be discouraged if you are not experiencing the benefits immediately. Losing weight and being healthy takes time. In order to do this, allow your body some time to start burning fat instead of glucose. It may take a few days or a couple of weeks, but be patient and don't bail ~~out~~ on the diet.

Tips for Successful Ketogenic Journey

I will be giving you some tips that will help you with your ketogenic diet challenge. The tips are kind of shortcuts to having a successful ketogenic diet.

Clear carbohydrates from your kitchen:

It is easier to stick to Keto if you have access to healthy ketogenic foods. Having Keto-unfriendly snacks in easy reach will only tempt you into falling prey to the carbohydrate concentrated foods in your pantry. Clean your kitchen of high-carbohydrate foods like pastry, bread, potatoes, soda, rice, and candy.

This will help in achieving and maintaining ketosis.

Have ketogenic snacks at hand:

Having to prepare a lot of homemade meals is a big challenge for people with a busy lifestyle. There is a solution for you: why not have ketogenic snacks instead whenever you are hungry, and you are not at home? You can buy ketogenic snacks like hard-boiled eggs, beef jerky, pre-cooked bacon, pre-made guacamole, and so on, or you can have them on the go. You can prepare a lot of them, and this will not allow you to buy carbohydrate-heavy snacks.

Buy a food scale:

This **pro-level tip** might sound surprising, but it is quite beneficial.

As it has been said, "Drops of water make an ocean." The amount of food you eat matters even to the tiniest form, especially when we are trying to stay under 50g of carbs per day. Buy a food scale to measure your food and make sure you are eating the appropriate serving sizes. Even the smallest amounts can make a big difference. For example, two extra tablespoons of almond butter turn out to be an additional 200 calories and 6 grams of carbohydrates.

You should read the nutrition labels and take note of the portion sizes used to calculate those values. Can you successfully lose weight without using a food scale? Absolutely! And you don't need to use the food scale all the way through your diet. Once you get a feel for portion sizes then, you can eyeball to measure it as you continue.

Exercise frequently:

We're not talking about running a marathon! Simple things will do the trick. Go two blocks further while walking your dog, taking the stairs rather than the elevator, and parking further away from your building will do the trick. Exercising allows your body to break down stored glycogen. It also helps you to get fit and healthy. It also helps you to maintain muscle mass and strength.

Try intermittent fasting:

This is one of the most effective tips that can get you right on track to achieving your fitness goals. It helps you get into ketosis and lose weight. This means that you do not eat anything that contains calories for a given period of time, usually 8-16 hours. When you stop eating for a short time, your body will start breaking down the excess glucose in your body obtained from consuming carbohydrates. You may also want to try the "5 and 2" method of fasting. You will consume no more than 500 calories on 2 non-consecutive days during the week.

Include coconut oil in your diet:

Coconut oil contains fats called medium-chain triglycerides which help you to get into ketosis quickly.

Unlike other fats, these MCTs are absorbed rapidly into the liver, where they are used for energy or converted into ketones.

Chapter 3: Ketogenic Diet and Weight-Loss

The ketogenic diet makes it possible for your body to break down its stored and unwanted fat. This is one of the major strategies used in bodybuilding to create muscle mass, even while decreasing overall body fat.

Most bodybuilders on the ketogenic diet regime set their everyday calorie intake to 20% more than their typical calorie level. This is not a set figure and should be adjusted on an individual basis. It is simply a guideline to point you in the right direction.

To consume the extra calories essential to the ketogenic diet program, you need to chow down on chicken, steak, fish, eggs, sausage, bacon, and protein shakes. You should consume 1.5g of extra fat for just about every gram of protein. Aim to eat upwards of five meals a day. Your muscles require more meals to grow. A key part of bodybuilding involves supplying your muscle tissue with nutrients.

If you are a serious bodybuilder or follow a strenuous workout routine, choose to load up on carbohydrates on a three-day cycle. On the third day, consume 1000 calories worth of carbs a minimum of two hours prior to your exercise routine for that day. You can choose from two alternatives of carb-loading. You can either eat anything that you would like or begin with higher glycemic carbs and then switch to lower glycemic carbs. If you decide against the targeted glycemic carbs approach, then you might want to stick to low-fat carbs. The reason behind the carb-loading is to enhance the glycogen within your muscle groups, which will enable you to endure an intense training session.

For instance, let us say you start by carb-loading on a Friday. By Sunday, your muscle tissues will have a substantial amount of glycogen in them. Sunday, then, is the day for strenuous exercise. It is optimal to only work out half of the body at this time with weights. Schedule your next exercise routine on Wednesday, and be sure to consume 1000 calories worth of carbs before your routine.

By Wednesday, your glycogen levels will likely be low, but the pre-workout carb load will allow you to work out intensely. This time you will perform exercises targeting the other half of your body.

The next exercise session should be Friday, at the beginning of the three-day cycle of loading up on carbohydrates.

This training session must be a complete overall body workout with 1-2 sets per workout completed until failure. Make barbell rows, bench presses, military presses, barbell/dumbbell curls, triceps pushdowns, squats, lunges, deadlifts, and reverse curls the focus of your training. The goal of this exercise session is to deplete your glycogen stores within the body completely. Nevertheless, keep cardio to a minimum. Ten-minute warm-ups in advance of each workout are okay but do not go overboard.

I'm on the ___ diet! You'll often hear that from your friends who are trying to slim down. There are thousands of diets out there.

Why should you try Keto over the others? You want to lose both weight and fat, right? Keto makes your body burn fat as its primary energy source. You don't have to starve yourself to lose weight with Keto. In fact, you should eat up to 20% more calories than normal. It's the kinds of foods that make the difference.

No bland, boring menus here, either.

The role of fats in a weight-loss program:

Fats contain twice the potential energy of carbohydrates and proteins. Fats protect organs and tissues and help maintain a constant temperature.

Weight Loss Tips:

Keep Your Carbs Very Low

This is the most significant thing while on keto. Keeping your carb intake to 50g or less helps to get the body into ketosis. It may take as long as two weeks to go into ketosis. Don't undo all your hard work by cheating.

Track Your Calories and Macros

This is very important while on a keto diet. Carbs are almost everywhere out there, and you need to keep track of all that you eat. Use the health app on your cellphone to help track carbs and calories.

Watch Your Electrolytes

Electrolytes need to be replenished frequently on the keto diet. Ensure that that you take enough potassium, magnesium, and sodium to curb excessive hunger, cramps, water retention, headaches, and cravings.

Be Patient:

Losing weight does not come overnight. You didn't gain all that weight overnight, and it won't come off overnight either. However, Keto is an effective way to lose weight and reduce body fat. When viewed as a lifestyle rather than a diet, Keto becomes rather easy. It's almost as easy as replacing sweet with savory!

Stress levels are also a factor in losing weight. When you are more stressed, the level of cortisol increases, which in turn causes weight gain or retention. And all to often we turn to "stress eating" when the pressure is on. Try deep breathing exercises instead. Chances are your cell phone has a stress tracker built in and will offer suggestions on stress relief.

Sleep and Rest:

Getting enough rest is critical to your overall health. Adequate sleep allows your body to recover. Most people require seven to nine hours of sleep for proper rest of the body each night.

Chapter 4: Meal Plan Ideas for Keto

Should I Try Keto?

Absolutely! With our hectic schedules these days, our diets have turned much more carbohydrate-heavy than in the past. Highly processed fast foods and super-sized portions have contributed to sky-high obesity rates. We all seem to be carrying a few extra pounds these days. The good news is that the Keto diet can help to shed those pounds quickly and safely.

And Keto doesn't have to cause a major lifestyle disruption. Almost any of your favorite foods can be made Keto-friendly.

Just substitute a low-carb alternative for the high-carb ones, and you're good to go.

Use almond or coconut flours instead of all-purpose flour. Use sweeteners in place of sugar. But do a little research first. Keto baking is rarely as simple as a 1:1 substitution of this for that. I would recommend finding and following Keto recipes rather than converting your favorite recipes. Some artificial sweeteners should not be used for baking, and some are significantly sweeter, or less sweet, than sugar. Others, such as Swerve, can substitute for sugar on a 1:1 ratio. Do a little experimenting to find the solutions that you like best.

The ideal meal plan for a ketogenic diet includes 5% carbs, 25% protein, and 70% fats. Intake of refined carbohydrates is a big no-no, as they are highly processed.

Refined carbohydrates contain high levels of sugar and empty carbs that will kick your body out of ketosis. Low-carb vegetables are highly recommended, and these include leafy vegetables such as spinach, lettuce, broccoli, cabbage, collard greens, kale, and cauliflower. When it comes to fats or oils, choosing healthy ones can reap benefits to one's health. Examples would include avocado, almonds, nuts, olives, organic coconut, peanut butter, sesame, and even dark chocolate can be healthy.

Remember to minimize hydrogenated oil or heated vegetable oils as they contain trans-fats that can clog the heart.

Because protein help repair tissues and cells, taking in protein is essential. The source of protein and cut choices should be taken into consideration as some parts are fattier and contain less protein. Examples of protein sources include grass-fed meats or wild games, free-range poultry, fish or seafood, shellfish, whole eggs, and whey protein powders.

The Keto diet may help those with pre-diabetes avoid significant blood sugar swings.

Some people find that a diet very low in carbohydrates feel lethargic (our muscles prefer to use glucose as fuel). If this is you, you can add a few slower acting carbohydrates in your such as berries, apples, beans, and oatmeal. Be sure to listen to your body and your doctor before making significant changes to your diet.

Low carb diets focus on lean meats, nuts, seeds, eggs, some dairy products, low-carb noodles, vegetables, and low-carbohydrate fruits such as berries. Lower carbohydrate plans can be beneficial for people who have not had success with other types of diets.

The added protein keeps you feeling full and staves off snack cravings. These plans can also be very beneficial for people with diabetes to help them maintain their level of sugar in the blood.

The Keto diet may reduce triglyceride levels and increase HDL cholesterol levels. People on a ketogenic diet should arrange to have their triglyceride and blood cholesterol levels monitored.

A Ketogenic diet generally results in rapid weight loss, which may help alleviate many conditions related to being overweight.

The Ketogenic Diet and Weightlifting

For fitness junkies on the ketogenic diet, it is recommended that you load up on carbohydrates on a three-day cycle. On the third day, consume 1000 calories worth of carbs at least two hours before your workout for that day.

You can pick between 2 options of carb-loading. You may either 1) eat anything that you need or 2) commence with high glycemic carbs and then switch to low glycemic carbs.

If you decide to eat anything that you want during this phase, then you need to stick to low-fat carbohydrates. The entire purpose behind the carb-loading is to increase the glycogen in your muscles, which will allow you to endure a powerful workout.

To get the extra calories required on the ketogenic diet, you will need to eat chicken, steak, fish, sausage, whole eggs, bacon, and protein shakes.

You want to consume 1.5g of fat for each gram of protein. Aim to eat upwards of five small meals each day. Your muscles need additional meals to grow.

The ketogenic diet allows your body to break down its stored fat. It is one of the main strategies employed in bodybuilding to create muscle mass while decreasing body fat. Most weightlifters on the ketogenic diet set their daily calorie consumption to twenty percent over their usual calorie level. This is not a set figure and can be changed on a personal basis. It is just a suggestion to get you moving in the correct direction.

Keto shows promise as an alternative remedy for cancer. The procedure of ketosis functions like this: glucose fuels every cell in our body, even the cancer cells. If we remove glucose, normal cells turn to ketone bodies to burn fats to survive- but not cancer cells.

They have no metabolic flexibility to do this. They will starve, thereby restricting their growth and therefore increasing the survival rates of cancer patients.

Keto has many benefits besides weight loss. The ketogenic diet was invented initially as a treatment for epilepsy. For people with type 2 diabetes, Keto can help change the way your body stores and uses energy. The diet's reduced carbs help reduce blood sugar spikes. And, as most type 2 diabetics are overweight, the weight loss on the Keto diet is a three-fold benefit.

The ease of unwrapping a candy bar have led to a glut of calories and easily burned glucose in our systems. There's no need for our bodies to burn fat because there is an over-abundance of glucose in the blood. So excess calories are stored as fat.

Keto is a safe, effective, and tasty way to turn that stored fat into energy.

Chapter 5: The Recipes

Breakfast Recipes

Spicy Scrambled Eggs and Bacon

Ingredients

4 strips of bacon

6 eggs, cracked into a bowl

2 tablespoons butter

1 Serrano chili, finely chopped

1/2 teaspoon salt

3/4 teaspoon onion powder

1/4 teaspoon black pepper

2 tablespoons sour cream

2 green onion stalks, sliced thin

Makes 2 servings; Net Carbs: 3.6 g per serving

Preparation:

Fry the bacon in a medium frying pan until it reaches the level of crispiness you desire, turning frequently. Remove bacon and set aside, reserve 1 tablespoon of the bacon fat. Place another medium frying pan on low heat and add the butter, reserved bacon fat, and chopped Serrano chili to it, sauté for 2 minutes.

While the chili is cooking, whisk together eggs, salt, onion powder, and black pepper in a medium bowl until smooth. Slowly pour into the warm pan with the cooked Serrano pepper. Wait until the bottom of the eggs begins to cook, and then use a silicone spatula to constantly stir and agitate the eggs until they are done to your satisfaction. Remove the eggs from the heat immediately.

Fold in the sour cream and green onion slices, making sure to distribute them evenly throughout the eggs.

Strawberry and Avocado Smoothie

Ingredients

1 cup ice

1 cup avocado

1 cup fresh or frozen strawberries

1 cup coconut milk beverage (unsweetened)

1/2 teaspoon vanilla extract

Zero carb sweetener of your choice (optional-to taste)

Makes 2 servings; Net Carbs: 6 g per serving

Preparation:

Put all the ingredients in a blender. Cover and blend at high speed until smooth.

Nut Granola

Ingredients

3/4 cup rough chopped pecans

3/4 cup rough chopped brazil nuts

1/2 cup rough chopped hazelnuts

1 tablespoon coconut oil

1 teaspoon cinnamon

1 teaspoon vanilla

1 tablespoon zero carb sweetener of your choice (optional-to taste)

Makes 4 servings; Net Carbs: 3 g per serving

Preparation:

Preheat oven to 285 F. Toss nuts and cinnamon together. Add melted coconut oil, vanilla, and sweetener (if desired). Toss again until nuts are well-coated. Line a shallow baking dish with parchment paper and spread nut mixture across it evenly. Bake 30-35 minutes until golden brown.

Cool.

Enjoy granola by itself or drenched in 1 cup cold, unsweetened almond milk (add 0.6 g net carbs) or 1 cup cold, unsweetened coconut milk (add 1 g net carbs).

Blueberry Muffins

Ingredients

3 cups almond flour

1/2 cup Xylitol or equivalent measurement of the zero carb sweetener of your choice

1/4 teaspoon Kosher salt

1-1/2 teaspoon baking powder

1/3 cup coconut oil

3 tablespoons unsalted butter

1/3 cup unsweetened almond milk

3 large egg

1/2 teaspoon vanilla extract

1 cup whole blueberries

Makes 12 servings; Net Carbs: 4 g per serving

Preparation:

Preheat the oven to 350°F and line muffin pan cups with liners.

Mix the flour, baking powder, salt and sweetener together in a large mixing bowl. Cut in the coconut oil in solid form and butter until lumps are no bigger than peas. In a separate bowl, combine milk, eggs, and vanilla. Add egg mixture to the flour mixture and combine until moistened. Fold in blueberries.

Divide batter evenly among the muffin cups and cook 25 minutes or until a toothpick inserted in muffin comes out clean.

Mini-ham Quiches

Ingredients

2 ounces Swiss cheese

4 slices of bacon, cooked

6 slices deli ham

5 eggs

1 tablespoon unsweetened almond milk

1/4 teaspoon salt

1/4 teaspoon pepper

1/4 teaspoon onion powder

non-stick cooking spray

Makes 6 servings; Net Carbs: 2 g per serving

Preparation:

Preheat the oven to 400 F. Dice the cheese and bacon.

In a small bowl, whisk together eggs, milk, salt, pepper, and onion powder.

Spray a 6-cup muffin pan and line each cup with one slice of the deli ham. Evenly distribute the cheese and bacon to each cup, and then fill each cup with the egg mixture until it fills each cup but be careful it does not overflow. You may want to use a measuring cup to help control the liquid as you fill them.

Bake for 20 minutes. Cool slightly before serving.

Crepes with Nut Butter and Whipped Cream

Ingredients

Nut Butter:

3/4 cup roasted, husked hazelnuts

2 tablespoons Xylitol or equivalent measurement of the zero carb sweetener of your choice

2 tablespoons cocoa powder

1/8 teaspoon salt

1/2 teaspoon vanilla extract

2 tablespoons coconut oil

Crepes:

1/2 cups almond flour

2 tablespoon Xylitol or equivalent measurement of the zero carb sweetener of your choice

4 ounces cream cheese brick

4 eggs

1/8 teaspoon salt

3 teaspoons salted butter

Whipped Cream:

1-1/2 cup heavy cream

3/4 teaspoon vanilla extract

3 tablespoon Xylitol or equivalent measurement of the zero carb sweetener of your choice

Makes 6 servings; Net Carbs: 6.55 g per 2-crepe serving

Preparation:

Note: You can store the crepes in the refrigerator after they have completely cooled (you might want to put parchment paper or plastic wrap between each one). You can also store the nut butter in the refrigerator for a couple of weeks. Once whipped, the whipping cream does not keep well, but you can keep it as a liquid in the fridge and then whip 1/4 cup per serving as you need it.

Finely ground nuts in a food processor. While continuing to grind, slowly add cocoa powder, salt, vanilla, and melted coconut oil until it reaches the desired consistency. If you want thinner nut butter, you can add up to 1 additional tablespoon of coconut oil for a total of 3 tablespoons.

Use a hand immersion blender to combine all the crepe ingredients except the butter in a 1-quart measuring cup or small pitcher. Using a crepe-maker or an 8" skillet, heat the pan over medium-low heat and use about ¼ teaspoon of butter to coat the pan. If you are using a crepe-maker, follow the provided instructions. Otherwise, pour 1/8 cup batter into the pan, quickly pick up the skillet, and swirl the pan to distribute the batter across the entire bottom of the pan. This may take some practice. It takes about 10 seconds for the crepe to finish cooking on one side. Once it is done, flip the crepe and cook another 10 seconds on the other side. Remove the crepe from the pan and place it on a plate. Continue making crepes until you are out of batter.

Whisk (by hand or with a stand mixer and the appropriate attachment) the cream, vanilla, and sweetener until stiff.

Place 1 crepe on a flat surface and spread 1 tablespoon of the nut butter on top of it. Spread 1 tablespoon of whipped cream on top of the nut butter and roll. When you have finished making the crepes, evenly distribute the left-over whipped cream on top of the crepe rolls.

Strawberry-Coconut Porridge

Ingredients

3/4 cup water

2 tablespoons ground flax seeds

2 tablespoons coconut flour

1/8 teaspoon kosher salt

1 egg, well-beaten

2 teaspoons butter

1 tablespoon coconut milk

1/4 cup strawberries

Greased loaf pans

Makes 1 serving; Net Carbs: 6.1 g per serving

Preparation:

In a medium saucepan, combine water, flax seeds, flour, and salt. Stirring frequently, heat on medium-high until the porridge thickens slightly. Remove from heat. Whisk in the egg, slowly until the porridge thickens and the egg is well-combined.

Serve in a bowl topped with the butter, coconut milk, and strawberries.

Ham, Egg, and Cheese Roll-ups

Ingredients

6 slices deli ham

6-1.3 ounce slices of cheddar cheese

4 eggs

1 tablespoon chives, finely sliced

1 tablespoon butter

1/4 teaspoon salt

1-1/8 teaspoon of black pepper

1/4 teaspoon of onion powder

Non-stick cooking spray

Toothpicks (soaked in water for 20 minutes)

Makes 3 servings; Net Carbs: 2.2 g per 2–roll serving

Preparation:

Preheat oven to 395 F.

Whisk together eggs, salt, onion powder, and black pepper in a medium bowl until smooth. Place a medium frying pan on low heat and melt the butter in it. Slowly pour the egg into the warm pan with the butter. Wait until the bottom of the eggs begins to cook, and then use a silicone spatula to constantly stir and agitate the eggs until they are done to your satisfaction. Remove the eggs from the heat immediately.

Lay out the slices of ham next to each other and top with a slice of cheese. Evenly distribute the eggs on top of each slice of cheese. Sprinkle chives on top of eggs.

Spray a small cooking dish with non-stick cooking spray. Roll the ham, egg, and cheese slices, using a soaked toothpick to secure the roll. Carefully transfer the rolls to the prepared cooking dish.

Bake 10 minutes until the ham is browned and its edges are slightly curled.

Lox Rolls

Ingredients

3 ounces cream cheese

1 teaspoon capers, very finely chopped

2 teaspoons chives, very finely sliced

1/2 tablespoon red onion, very finely chopped

1/2 teaspoon grated lemon peel

3 ounces boneless lox (or smoked salmon if you prefer it)

Toothpicks

Makes 2 servings; Net Carbs: 2 g per 4-piece serving

Preparation:

Use a hand immersion blender to combine the cream cheese, capers, chives, red onion, and lemon peel. Cut the lox into 1/2-ounce pieces (you should have a total of 8 pieces that are about the same size). Spread the cream cheese mixture on each piece evenly distributing it between pieces.

Roll the lox around the cream cheese and secure with a toothpick.

Spinach Omelet in a Mug

Ingredients:

2 eggs

2 tablespoons heavy cream

2 tablespoons finely grated cheddar cheese

1/8 teaspoon garlic powder

1/8 teaspoon Kosher salt

1/8 teaspoon black pepper

1/2 cup fresh spinach

Makes 1 serving; Net Carbs: 2.3 g per serving

Preparation:

Whisk together eggs, cream, cheddar cheese, garlic, salt, and black pepper in a medium bowl until smooth. Place spinach leaves in a 10-ounce mug. Carefully pour the egg mixture over the spinach, being sure to pour slowly.

Microwave on high for 1-1/2 minutes until the eggs are thoroughly cooked.

Lunch Recipes

Spinach Pecan Salad

Ingredients:

6 cups spinach

1/4 cup red onions, sliced thinly

1/2 cup pecan halves

1/2 cup crumbled feta cheese

1/4 cup apple cider vinegar

1/4 cup olive oil

1/4 teaspoon Kosher salt

1/4 teaspoon pepper

Makes 4 servings; Net Carbs: 3 g per serving

Preparation:

Note: Salad and vinaigrette can be prepared a day in advance as long as they are not combined until serving. Vinaigrette should be whisked before combining.

Toast pecans in a 450 F oven for 3 minutes and then set aside to cool.

Whisk vinegar, olive oil, salt, and pepper in a small bowl until blended.

In a separate large bowl toss spinach, pecans, and feta.

Drizzle with vinaigrette on top and toss again.

Enjoy your meal.

Chicken Strips & Cauliflower Bites

Ingredients:

Chicken Strips:

2 eggs

2 teaspoons Dijon mustard

1 teaspoon salt

1 teaspoon black pepper

1-1/2 cup finely grated (fresh) Parmesan cheese

1/4 cup almond flour

4 tablespoons cooking oil

1-pound boneless, skinless chicken breasts cut into 8 tenders or 8 pre-cut tenders

Cauliflower Bites:

12 ounces (about 1/2 a large head) cauliflower

4 egg yolks

3/4 cup almond flour

3/4 cup finely grated (fresh) Parmesan cheese

1 teaspoon garlic powder

1/2 teaspoon salt

1/2 teaspoon cayenne pepper (optional)

3/4 cup butter

Makes 4 servings; Chicken Strip Net Carbs: 3 g per 2-piece serving; Cauliflower Bites Net Carbs: 7 g per serving; Meal Net Carbs: 10 g per serving

Preparation:

Whisk together eggs, brown mustard, salt, and pepper. Toss together the cheese and almond flour.

Heat cooking oil on high until hot. Dip each tender first in the egg mixture and then in the cheese mixture. Place them in the oil to cook until done, approximately 5 minutes. Remove from oil and place on a paper towel.

Break cauliflower into florets and place in a skillet with about 1/4-inch of water. Bring to a simmer, and then reduce heat and cover for 8 minutes. Drain off any remaining water and set aside to cool.

Whisk together the egg yolks, garlic, salt, and cayenne pepper (if desired) in a small bowl. Toss the bread crumbs and cheese together in a separate bowl. Melt the butter in a skillet over medium-high heat.

Carefully place the cauliflower florets into the egg yolk mixture
a few at a time, making sure they are well coated. Then
transfer them to the bread crumb mixture using a slotted
spoon and toss them to coat. Transfer them to the skillet with
the butter and cook until brown, approximately 4 minutes.

Hot Curried Pumpkin Soup

Ingredients:

1 (15-ounce) can pumpkin

1/4 cup coconut oil

1 cup onion, chopped

1 clove minced garlic

3 cups chicken broth

1 teaspoon curry powder

1/2 teaspoon salt

1/2 teaspoon coriander

1/2 teaspoon crushed red pepper flakes

1/2 teaspoon cinnamon

1/2 teaspoon fresh grated ginger

1 cup coconut milk

1/4 small apple cubed

3 slices bacon, cooked

6 teaspoons sour cream

Zero carb sweetener of your choice (optional-to taste)

Makes 6 1-cup servings; Net Carbs: 3.1 g per serving

Preparation:

Heat the coconut oil until melted in a Dutch oven. Sauté the onions and garlic in the pot until the onions become translucent, approximately 5 minutes. Add the vegetable broth, salt, and seasonings. Cook on medium heat until the mixture comes to a gentle boil, and then cover and cook an additional 15-20 minutes, stirring occasionally.

Whisk together the coconut milk and pumpkin and then add this mixture to the pot. Continue cooking for another 5 minutes. Taste the soup to determine if it is sweet/spicy enough for you. You can add zero carb sweetener to make the soup sweet and/or add additional curry or red pepper to increase the heat. Once it is adjusted, use a hand immersion blender to process the soup until it is smooth.

Divide the apple cubes into six bowls. Pour 1 cup of soup in each bowl and garnish with 1 teaspoon sour cream and 1/2 slice of crumbled bacon.

Hot and Spicy Thai Beef Salad

Ingredients:

4 ounces lean sirloin steak

2 teaspoons olive oil

1/4 teaspoon rice vinegar

1/8 teaspoon salt

1/8 teaspoon pepper

1 clove garlic

1/2 teaspoon zero carb chili paste

1/2 teaspoon lime juice

1-1/2 ounce spinach

1 ounce coleslaw mix

1 ounce cucumber, chopped

2 teaspoons olive oil

1/4 teaspoon rice vinegar

1/4 teaspoon salt

1/4 teaspoon pepper

1/8 teaspoon curry powder

Makes 1 serving; Net Carbs: 4 g per serving

Preparation:

The night before: Cut the steak into thin strips. In a plastic baggie, combine 2 teaspoons of the olive oil, salt, pepper, garlic, chili paste, and lime juice. Add the meat to this bag of marinade and seal the bag. Allow the meat to marinate in your refrigerator 6-24 hours.

After the steak has marinated: Toss the spinach, coleslaw mix, and cucumber together. Combine the remaining olive oil, vinegar, salt, pepper, and curry powder and add this oil mixture to the salad. Tossing lightly. Place salad on serving plate.

Cook steak in a small skillet over high heat until it reaches your preferred level of doneness. Flip half-way through cooking. Place steak on top of salad and serve.

Mushroom Pizza Bites

Ingredients:

4 whole portabella mushroom caps with the stems removed

4-1/2 ounces mozzarella cheese cut into 4 even slices

8 slices pepperoni

4 slices 1/4" thick from a large tomato

1/2 teaspoon salt

1/4 teaspoon pepper

2 teaspoons oregano

1 tablespoon basil

1 clove garlic

2 tablespoons olive oil

Makes 4 servings; Net Carbs: 5.2 g per single mushroom serving

Preparation:

Preheat broiler.

Place Portobello mushroom caps upside down on a broiler-safe pan. Toss stir the oil and garlic together in a small, spouted measuring cup and drizzle oil mixture over the mushrooms. Place one slice of mozzarella on top of each mushroom and then top that with two slices of pepperoni and a tomato slice. Sprinkle oregano, basil, salt, and pepper on top of the tomato slices.

Broil 6-8 minutes being careful not to overcook. The cheese should be melted.

Sriracha Chicken Fried Rice

Ingredients:

3/4 cup cauliflower rice

2 tablespoons soy sauce

1/8 teaspoon black pepper

1/4 teaspoon garlic powder

1 egg

1 tablespoon olive oil

4 ounces chicken breast, chopped into 1" cubes

1/4 teaspoon salt

1/4 teaspoon black pepper

1-1/2 ounce broccoli, chopped

1/2 tablespoon Sriracha sauce

1/2 tablespoon green onions, chopped

Makes 1 servings; Net Carbs: 7 g per serving

Preparation:

In a medium skillet over medium-high heat, combine cauliflower rice, soy sauce, 1/8 teaspoon black pepper, and garlic powder. Cook until rice is browned and slightly crispy. Whisk the egg in a small bowl and add it into the rice while stirring to scramble it. Once the egg part of the mixture is cooked, transfer it to a bowl.

Add the oil to the skillet and return it to medium-high heat. Add the chicken to the oil and toss to coat with the oil. Season with salt and pepper. Cook until chicken is browned.

Add the broccoli to the chicken and cook until tender. Add Sriracha sauce and toss to coat. Remove from heat. Add the chicken mixture to the bowl on top of the rice. Garnish with the green onion.

Enjoy your meal.

Taco Bowl

Ingredients:

1 teaspoon olive oil

10 ounces 90% lean ground beef or ground turkey

1/2 teaspoon salt

1/4 teaspoon black pepper

1/2 teaspoon onion powder

1/4 teaspoon ground cumin

1/4 teaspoon cayenne pepper

1-1/2 cup cauliflower rice

4-1/2 ounces avocado, sliced evenly into 9 slices

3 teaspoons cilantro, finely chopped

9 tablespoons shredded cheddar cheese

Makes 3 servings; Net Carbs: 3 g per serving

Preparation:

Note: The extra bowls can be stored in the refrigerator for up to three days.

In a large skillet, cook the ground meat, olive oil, salt, pepper, cumin, cayenne, and onion powder on high until meat is fully cooked, approximately 8 minutes. Using a slotted spoon, distribute the meat equally into three containers or bowls. Discard any liquid that is remaining in the skillet.

Return the skillet to medium heat. Add the rice cauliflower and cook until slightly browned. Equally distribute the rice into the three containers next to the meat. Each container will receive about 1/2 cup of rice. Sprinkle the 1 teaspoon of cilantro over the rice and meat in each container, and add 3 slices of avocado and 3 tablespoons of cheese to each.

Sesame Crusted Tuna

Ingredients:

2 tuna steaks 4-1/2 ounces each steak

1/8 teaspoon salt

1/8 teaspoon ground ginger

2 tablespoons whole sesame seeds

2 teaspoons olive oil

2 teaspoons soy sauce

3 tablespoons store mayonnaise

1 teaspoon Sriracha sauce or your favorite zero carb hot chili sauce

Makes 2 servings; Net Carbs: 2 g per serving

Preparation:

Place the tuna steaks on a flat, clean surface and sprinkle with salt and ginger. Place the olive oil in a skillet over medium heat.

Place the sesame seeds on a plate and gently press all sides of
the tuna steaks into the seeds to coat the steaks. Once coated,
add the soy sauce to the oil and cook the steaks in the mixture,
covered, until the desired level of doneness is reached. Flip
steaks at least once half-way through cooking. Seeds should be
at least golden in color when the steaks are done.

Whisk together the mayonnaise and hot sauce. Serve each of
the steaks with half of the mayonnaise sauce.

Chicken and Bacon Salad

Ingredients:

4 slices bacon, cooked, cut into 1" slices

1 cup rotisserie chicken, cut in 1" cubes

1/2 cup cheddar cheese, grated

2 teaspoons chives, finely chopped

2 scallions each 3" long, thinly sliced

2 tablespoons sour cream

2 tablespoons olive oil

2 cups Romaine lettuce, chopped

1/8 teaspoon salt

1/8 teaspoon black pepper

Makes 2 servings; Net Carbs: 3 g per serving

Preparation:

Toss lettuce, scallions, and chives. Add olive oil, chicken,
bacon, and cheese. Toss again to evenly distribute. Sprinkle

cheese and salt and pepper on top. Spoon the sour cream on to the top. Split evenly into two bowls and serve.

Asparagus Soup

Ingredients:

2 tablespoons butter

1 clove garlic, minced

1 tablespoon red onion, minced

1/4 teaspoon sea salt

1/8 teaspoon black pepper

1-1/2 cup asparagus chopped into 1-1/2" pieces

3 cups vegetable stock

1/3 cup heavy cream

Makes 4 servings; Net Carbs: 3.6 g per serving

Preparation:

Combine butter, onion, and garlic in a medium saucepan. Add asparagus to the pan and continue to sauté 4 more minutes. Remove the tips of the asparagus from the pan and set aside. Add the vegetable stock, salt, and pepper to the pan and simmer for another 6 minutes. Use a hand immersion stick blender to blend the soup until smooth. Return add the asparagus tips and the cream into soup. Once the soup is heated through, divide it evenly into four bowls.

Dinner Recipes

Salmon with Dill Sauce and Roasted Asparagus

Ingredients:

Salmon:

2 boneless, raw, six-ounce salmon filets

1 tablespoon olive oil

1/4 teaspoon salt

1/4 teaspoon black pepper

1/2 teaspoon parsley

4 lemon slices each 1/4" thick

1-1/2 tablespoons butter

1/4 cup onions, finely diced

1 clove garlic, minced

1 cup heavy cream

1/8 teaspoon salt

1/4 teaspoon black pepper

1/2 teaspoon lemon zest

2 tablespoons dill

1/2 tablespoon Greek yogurt

Non-stick cooking spray

Roasted Asparagus:

1/2 pound asparagus, ends removed

2 tablespoons olive oil

1/4 lemon, zest and juice

1 teaspoon Kosher salt

1/8 teaspoon black pepper

1/4 ounce fresh parmesan cheese, grated finely

Makes 2 servings; Salmon Net Carbs: 7 g per 10-piece serving; Asparagus Net Carbs: 2 g per serving; Meal Net Carbs: 9 g per serving

Preparation:

Preheat oven to 375 F.

Spray a large piece of foil with non-stick cooking spray. Place salmon, skin side down, in the center of the foil. Rub olive oil on the filets and then sprinkle each evenly with salt, pepper, and parsley. Place 2 slices of lemon on each filet. Fold the foil over and seal it securely. Place the foil packet in a baking dish and bake for about 20 minutes until salmon is desired doneness.

Place asparagus in a single layer on a shallow baking sheet. Drizzle olive oil and then the lemon juice evenly over the asparagus. Sprinkle salt, pepper, and zest over the top of the asparagus. Place in the oven for about 15 minutes until desired tenderness is achieved. Sprinkle parmesan over the asparagus as soon as it is removed from the oven. Divide evenly between two plates.

Sauté butter, onions, and garlic in a medium skillet over medium-low heat until onions are translucent. Add the heavy cream, pepper, salt, dill, and zest. Simmer uncovered for 3-4 minutes, and then remove from heat. Slightly cool and add the Greek yogurt. Place one salmon filet on each plate and divide sauce equally between them.

Swedish Meatballs

Ingredients:

4 tablespoons butter

1 medium, white onion, chopped

1 lb. ground beef

1/4 cup crushed pork rinds

1/2 teaspoon salt

1/2 teaspoon ground black pepper

1/4 teaspoon allspice

1/4 teaspoon nutmeg

1/4 teaspoon garlic powder

1 egg

1 teaspoon Dijon mustard

3/4 teaspoon arrowroot powder

2 tablespoons cold water

1 cup beef broth

1/2 cup heavy cream

16 ounces Tofu and Shirataki noodles

Makes 4 servings; Net Carbs: 6.5 g per serving

Preparation:

Melt a tablespoon of butter in large skillet and sauté onion in it over medium heat. Combine beef, pork rind, beaten egg, onion, salt, spices, and 2 tablespoons heavy cream in a large bowl. Mix thoroughly. Divide into 16 equal sized meatballs. Melt the rest of the butter in the skillet over medium heat and add the meatballs. Cook until meatballs are cooked through, moving them so they brown on all sides as they cook, about 15 minutes. Remove from heat and transfer to a plate.

Add the broth, remaining cream, and mustard to the pan and simmer on low, scraping the bottom for flavor. Mix the arrowroot powder and water in a small measuring cup to make a slurry and add it to the sauce. Continue simmering on low until the sauce is the desired thickness.

Return the meatballs to the sauce and simmer a couple minutes longer. Cover and remove from heat.

Prepare noodles according to package directions, draining well. Evenly divide the noodles between four plates. Then cover each bed of noodles with an equal amount of sauce and four meatballs.

BBQ Chicken Wings with Loaded Cauliflower Mash

Ingredients:

BBQ Chicken Rub:

2 teaspoons garlic powder

2 teaspoons onion powder

2 teaspoons gourmet smoked paprika

1 tablespoon Xylitol or equivalent measurement of the zero carb sweetener of your choice

1 teaspoon cayenne pepper

1/2 teaspoon ground ginger

1/2 teaspoon cumin

1/2 teaspoon cinnamon

1/2 teaspoon coriander

1/4 teaspoon salt

1/4 teaspoon black pepper

BBQ Chicken:

2 pounds skin-on, chicken wings

2 teaspoons coconut oil

3 teaspoons tomato puree

1 tablespoon coconut oil

1/2 cup chicken stock

1 tablespoon butter

1 teaspoon mustard

Loaded Cauliflower Mash:

1 pound cauliflower

1 tablespoon butter

1/2 cup sour cream

1 clove garlic, minced

1/8 teaspoon salt

1/4 teaspoon black pepper

2 slices bacon, cooked, and chopped into small pieces

1/2 cup cheddar cheese, shredded

1 tablespoon chives, chopped

Makes 4 servings; BBQ Chicken Net Carbs: 2 g per 1/2-pound serving; Cauliflower Mash Net Carbs: 4 .6 g per serving; Meal Net Carbs: 6.6 g per serving

Preparation:

Preheat oven to 375 F.

Make rub by combining all the ingredients for it and mixing until well-blended. Place half (about 6 teaspoons) into a small saucepan. Grease a baking dish with 2 teaspoons coconut oil, using all of it. Arrange wings in the dish in a single layer and sprinkle remaining rub on top, rubbing it into the meat. Bake wings in oven for 40 minutes.

Steam the cauliflower using the microwave by placing it in a microwave safe bowl with three tablespoons of water and covering. Microwave on high about 5 minutes adding 2 minutes at a time after that until cauliflower is soft and easy to break apart. Immediately drain any excess water and allow to sit in colander for 5 minutes. Transfer to food processor with butter, garlic, sour cream, salt, and pepper. Process until desired consistency.

Transfer mash to an oven safe baking dish. Evenly sprinkle bacon and cheddar over the top.

When the chicken comes out of the oven, place the remaining coconut oil , butter, tomato puree, and mustard into the pan with the rub. Over low heat, whisk the sauce together, slowly adding in the stock. Once the stock is the correct consistency, remove from heat and pour over chicken immediately. Place mash in oven and return chicken and sauce to the oven for another 20-25 minutes.

Divide chicken wings onto four plates with about 1/2 pound of wings on each and divide the mash evenly between the plates.

Pot Roast

Ingredients:

48 ounces boneless, lean chuck roast

2 teaspoons Kosher salt

1-1/2 teaspoons coconut oil

5 large stalks celery

1 cup carrots, chopped

1/2 cup onions, chopped

4 cups beef broth

3 teaspoons thyme, fresh, chopped

1/4 teaspoon black pepper

Makes 6 servings; Net Carbs: 3 g per serving

Preparation:

In a stock pot over medium-high heat, melt the coconut oil.

Season the beef with one teaspoon of salt on each side and place it in the pan to brown for approximately 5 minutes on each side. Add all the other ingredients to the pot and simmer, covered, on low heat for approximately 2 hours until meat is cooked to desired doneness. Evenly divide the vegetables and meat between six plates.

Garlic-Rosemary Pork Chops with Roasted Brussels Sprouts

Ingredients:

Pork Chops:

2 pounds bone-in pork chops, center cut (ideally there would be 4 chops that each are about 1/2 pound)

1-1/2 teaspoons Kosher salt

1/2 teaspoon black pepper

4 tablespoons fresh rosemary, broken into 2" sprigs

4 cloves garlic, whole

4 tablespoons salted butter

2-1/2 tablespoons apple cider vinegar

1-1/2 tablespoons ghee (clarified butter)

Brussels Sprouts:

12-1/2 ounces Brussels sprouts

4 slices bacon, raw, chopped

2 tablespoons capers

1 tablespoon olive oil

1/8 teaspoon sea salt

1/8 teaspoon black pepper

Makes 4 servings; Pork Chops Net Carbs: 1 g per serving; Brussels Sprouts Net Carbs: 4 g per serving; Meal Net Carbs: 5 g per serving

Preparation:

Preheat the oven to 400 F.

Slice Brussels sprouts in half and arrange in a single layer in a baking dish. Toss with bacon, olive oil, salt, and pepper. Bake 15 minutes.

Sprinkle the pork chops with the salt and pepper on both sides. Melt the ghee in a large skillet on low, then add the pork chops. Sear 5-7 minutes on each side before flipping. After you flip, add butter, rosemary, and garlic to the skillet. As the butter melts, spoon it over the chops. Remove the chops and add the vinegar to the skillet. Scrape the pan as you mix the vinegar, seasoning, and butter.

Remove Brussels sprouts from oven. Add capers and toss again. Return to oven for another 5-8 minutes until bacon is crisp.

Divide into 4 equal portions and place on plates with chops.
Drizzle butter mixture from pan over each chop.

Chicken Cordon Bleu with Garlic Keto Bread

Ingredients:

Chicken Cordon Bleu:

24 ounces boneless, skinless chicken breast

1/2 teaspoon salt

1/2 teaspoon black pepper

4 slices deli ham

4-1/2 ounces Swiss cheese, sliced

12 slices bacon, raw

4 teaspoons olive oil

1/2 cup shredded parmesan

2 tablespoons parsley

Bread:

1 cup almond flour

1 teaspoon double-acting baking powder

1/8 teaspoon Kosher salt

1/4 teaspoon xanthan gum

1/2 cup butter

2 tablespoons coconut oil

6 eggs, separated

Garlic Butter:

1 clove garlic, minced

1/4 cup finely grated (fresh) Parmesan cheese

4 tablespoons butter

Makes 4 servings; Chicken Cordon Bleu Net Carbs: 2 g per 2-piece serving; Garlic Toast Net Carbs: 4.6 g per serving; Meal Net Carbs: 6.6 g per serving

Preparation:

Preheat oven to 375 F.

Begin by whipping together the garlic, parmesan cheese, and butter to make the garlic butter. Set aside to keep it soft and at room temperature.

In a food processor, combine the dry parts of the bread recipe: flour, baking powder, salt, and xanthan gum as well as the fats: butter and coconut oil. When a dough forms, add in the egg yolks. Blend the egg whites until they reach a soft peak stage. Carefully fold these into the batter and then pour into a parchment lined loaf pan that is greased on the sides with butter. Bake 25- 30 minutes and allow to cool completely.

Butterfly chicken breasts and pound to 1/2-inch thickness using a meat tenderizer. Sprinkle salt and pepper evenly over inside portion of the chicken. Place one slice of ham on each chicken breast and arrange Swiss cheese in a single layer over ham. Fold the chicken to return it to its original form, being careful to keep the ham and cheese on the inside of the fold. Wrap each breast in bacon, using 3 slices to evenly wrap each. Keep the ends of the bacon underneath the chicken to prevent it from unwrapping.

Heat olive oil in a large skillet on medium high heat. Add wrapped chicken and cover. Cook chicken for about 5 minutes on each side or until the chicken is cooked through and juices are clear. Sprinkle with parmesan cheese and cover again until the cheese melts, about 45 seconds.

Preheat the broiler. Slice the cooled bread in half length-wise and then slice each half in half again parallel to the counter. Butter the bread with one-fourth of the garlic butter and place face up on a baking pan. Broil 2 minutes until butter and cheese have melted.

Keto Pepperoni Pizza

Ingredients:

3-1/2 cups shredded mozzarella, divided

2 tablespoons cream cheese

1 egg

3/4 cup almond flour

1 teaspoon Italian seasoning

1/3 cup Rao's Marinara

1/4 cup sliced pepperoni

Makes 8 slices; Net Carbs: 4 g per slice

Preparation:

Preheat oven to 425 F.

Mix together cream cheese and only 2 cups of the mozzarella
in a microwave safe bowl. Place in the microwave on high for a
minute. Stir. Return to the microwave for 30 more seconds and
stir again. Continue alternating stirring and mircowaving until
the cheese comes together. Add flour, egg, and Italian
seasoning to the cheese mixture.

Pour the dough onto a large piece of parchment paper. Place an equally large piece on top of the dough and roll the dough into a circle in the shape of a 12" pizza crust. Carefully remove the top piece of parchment. Transfer the dough and bottom parchment sheet to a pizza pan.

Bake 10 minutes until lightly golden brown. Carefully flip pizza crust and bake another 3 minutes.

Remove crust from oven and evenly spread the marinara over it. Sprinkle on the remaining mozzarella and evenly distribute the pepperoni slices.

Once assembled, bake an additional 10 minutes. Slice into 8 even slices.

Firecracker Shrimp with Bacony Broccoli

Ingredients:

Firecracker Shrimp:

20 large shrimp (uncooked, peeled, deveined)

4 tablespoons Sriracha hot sauce

4 teaspoons rice vinegar

1/4 cup soy sauce

1 tablespoon lime juice

1/2 teaspoon black pepper

2 teaspoons sesame seeds

1 clove garlic, minced

Bacony Broccoli:

 1 slice bacon

1/2 tablespoon butter

1 cup broccoli, chopped

1/8 teaspoon salt

1/8 teaspoon black pepper

1/4 teaspoon ginger

1/8 teaspoon garlic powder

Makes 2 servings; Shrimp Net Carbs: 5 g per 10-piece serving; Bacony Broccoli Net Carbs: 2 g per serving; Meal Net Carbs: 7 g per serving

Preparation:

At least one hour before: In a bowl, combine shrimp, Sriracha, rice vinegar, soy sauce, lime juice, pepper, sesame seeds, and garlic. Cover and allow the shrimp to marinate in your refrigerator 1-12 hours.

Right before eating: Cook the bacon to desired doneness in a medium skillet. Set aside to cool. Melt butter into the bacon grease over medium-low heat and add the broccoli. Cover and cook until tender, approximately 5 minutes. Add salt, pepper, ginger, and garlic powder and toss until well mixed. Chop bacon into small pieces and return them to the pan. Remove from heat and divide evenly between two plates.

Empty the shrimp and all the marinade into a large skillet and cook over medium heat, being sure to flip the shrimp at least once, half-way through cooking. When sauce is slightly reduced and shrimp is cooked through, remove from heat and divide evenly between the two plates.

Beefy Chili

Ingredients:

2-1/2 pounds ground beef

1/2 large white onion

4 cloves garlic, minced

30 ounces canned, diced tomatoes with liquid

6 ounces canned tomato paste

4 ounces canned green chilies with liquid

1/4 cup chili powder

2 tablespoons Worcestershire sauce

2 tablespoons cumin

1 tablespoons dried oregano

 2 teaspoons sea salt

1 teaspoon black pepper

Serving size is one cup of cooked chili; Net Carbs: 10 g per serving

Preparation:

Cook the onion, garlic, and ground beef in a large skillet over medium-high heat for about 15 minutes until the onions are translucent and the beef is browned, stirring to break beef into small pieces.

Place beef in a slow cooker and add the remaining ingredients. Mix well.

Set the slow cooker to low and cook 6-8 hours or to high and cook 3-4 hours.

Turkey Casserole

Ingredients:

1 pound skinless, boneless turkey breast, chopped into 1" cubes

1 tablespoon olive oil

3 cups broccoli

3 tablespoons water

1 tablespoon butter, unsalted

1 clove garlic, minced

3/4 cup chicken broth

2 tablespoons parmesan cheese, finely grated

1 cup cheddar cheese, finely grated

3/4 cup cream cheese spread

1 ounce almonds, finely ground

1/4 teaspoon sea salt

1/8 teaspoon black pepper

Makes 4 servings; Net Carbs: 8 g per serving

Preparation:

Preheat the oven to 400 F.

In a medium skillet, combine the olive oil and turkey and stir-fry until turkey is browned on all sides. Remove from heat, and set pan aside.

Steam the broccoli using the microwave by placing it in a microwave safe bowl with three tablespoons of water and covering. Microwave on high about 3 minutes until broccoli is tender. Immediately drain any excess water and toss together with the turkey in the skillet.

Heat butter, garlic, and broth in a small saucepan over low heat. When hot, add cream cheese and cheddar cheese, and mix well until the cheese has melted. Bring sauce to a simmer for two minutes until slightly thick.

Toss almonds and parmesan together. Spray a cooking dish with non-stick cooking spray. Place turkey mixture in the cooking dish. Pour cheese sauce on top. Sprinkle with almond-cheese mixture. Place dish in oven and bake 20-25 minutes

until heated through and bubbling. Top should be golden
brown.

Dessert Recipes

Creamy Raspberry Mousse

Ingredients:

1/2 cup raspberries

1/3 cup full fat coconut milk

2-4 tablespoons Xylitol or equivalent measurement of the zero
carb sweetener of your choice

3 tablespoons cocoa powder

2/3 cup heavy whipping cream

Makes 2 servings; Net Carbs: 5.3 g per serving

Preparation:

In a small saucepan, bring sweetener, cocoa, and coconut milk
to a simmer. Immediately remove from heat and cool, in an ice
bath if possible, mixing while it cools. In a separate, chilled

bowl, whisk heavy whipping cream to stiff peaks. Fold cream
mixture into chocolate mixture. Transfer equally to two serving
glasses and chill covered for a minimum of 1 hour, but 12
hours is best. Garnish with 1/4-cup raspberries on each.

Enjoy your dessert.

Pecan Pie

Ingredients:

1-1/4 cups almond meal or almond flour for finer consistency crust

1/4 cup flax seeds, ground

2 teaspoons ground cinnamon

1/2 cup coconut oil

1/8 teaspoon salt

2/3 cup Xylitol or equivalent measurement of the zero carb sweetener of your choice

2 tablespoons unsalted almond butter

1 cup pecans, chopped

1 teaspoon vanilla extract

3/4 cup almond milk

1-3 tablespoons warm water

Makes 8 servings; Net Carbs: 3 g per slice

Preparation:

In a food processor, combine almond meal, flax, 1 teaspoon cinnamon, and salt. Once well mixed, add 2 tablespoons coconut oil and pulse to create crumb mixture. Slowly add warm water just until a dough ball forms. Press dough evenly into a 7" tart pan. Place in fridge until firm, at least 20 minutes.

In a medium saucepan, combine 1/2 cup of almond milk, 1/4 cup of coconut oil and half the sweetener. Bring mixture to a boil while stirring, and then reduce the heat and simmer.

Preheat oven to 360 F.

Once the filling is simmering, add the remaining milk, cinnamon, almond butter, and vanilla to the filling, stirring well. Continue simmering until filling is sticky and brown. Remove from heat. The filling should resemble melted caramel. Stir in the pecans immediately. Spoon filling into the chilled tart shell, spreading it evenly as you go.

Bake 30-35 minutes until tart is cooked through. Allow to cool completely before cutting into 8 even slices and removing from the tin.

Pumpkin Pie Mini-Muffins

Ingredients:

1/2 cups canned pumpkin puree

4 teaspoons Xylitol or equivalent measurement of the zero carb sweetener of your choice

5 ounces cream cheese

1 egg

1/2 teaspoon cinnamon

1/2 teaspoon cinnamon

1-1/4 teaspoon pumpkin pie spice

Makes 6 servings; Net Carbs: 4 g per 2-mini-muffin serving

Preparation:

Preheat oven to 350 F.

Use the paddle attachment for your mixer and combine the sweetener and cream cheese until well-blended and smooth, approximately 4 minutes. Add in the pumpkin puree and eggs, again combining until no lumps remain and the batter is uniform. Finally, add in the spices. Line 12 mini-muffin cups with mini-muffin liners. Fill each with an equal amount of batter, leaving only 1/8-inch at the top for rising. When all cups are filled gently tap the tray against the counter to flatten the batter.

Bake for about 15 minutes and then reduce the heat to 300 F and cook an additional 10 minutes or until a toothpick inserted in the center comes out clean. Allow muffins to cool completely before attempting to remove liners or serve.

Lemon Cheesecake

Ingredients:

1-1/2 cups almond meal or almond flour for finer consistency crust

1 tablespoon butter

1 tablespoon coconut butter

3/4 cup Xylitol or equivalent measurement of the zero carb sweetener of your choice

1/8 teaspoon salt

14 ounces cream cheese

3/4 cup heavy cream

1 tablespoon lemon juice

1 tablespoon lemon zest

Makes 8 servings; Net Carbs: 5 g per slice

Preparation:

Pulse almond meal, butter, coconut oil. 1/4 cup sweetener, and salt in a food processor until crumbly. Press crust mixture firmly and evenly into a 6" springform pan. Place pan in the fridge to chill.

If you use Xylitol as your sweetener (or other course sweeteners), place the remaining amount in your food processor and process until very fine and powdery. Then add it to a mixing bowl containing the cream cheese, lemon juice, and 1/2 tablespoon of the zest, and cream it until well blended. Whisk cream into the cream cheese mixture until thick and smooth.

Remove the chilled crust from the fridge and smooth the cheesecake mixture over the top of it evenly. (Do not remove the edge of the springform pan, yet.) Place the whole cheesecake back in the refrigerator and chill another 5-18 hours. Remove the springform edge, sprinkle with remaining zest, and slice into 8 even pieces.

Crème Brule

Ingredients:

4 egg yolks

2 cups heavy cream

1/2 cup Xylitol or equivalent measurement of the zero carb sweetener of your choice

2 teaspoons vanilla extract

Makes 4 servings; Net Carbs: 4 g per serving

Preparation:

Preheat oven to 325 F.

In a small saucepan, heat cream until just before it simmers. Whisk together the egg yolks, sweetener, and vanilla in a small bowl until well-blended. Slowly add the egg mixture to the cream, making sure to vigorously whisk the cream while adding it.

Remove cream from heat and evenly divide the mixture between four, oven-proof ramekins. Place the ramekins into a baking pan with enough hot water in it to come up the sides of the ramekins by about 1". Bake in the water bath for about 1 hour.

Chill for at least 1 hour until firm. Use a culinary torch to brown the top if preferred.

Blueberry Streusel Bars

Ingredients:

6 tablespoons salted butter, melted

2 cups almond flour

1/2 cup Xylitol or equivalent measurement of the zero carb sweetener of your choice (if sweetener is not as fine as powdered/confectioners/icing sugar, be sure to process it in a food processor first)

1/8 teaspoon Kosher salt

1/2 teaspoon cinnamon

1-1/2 cup frozen, unsweetened blueberries

1/4 cup Xylitol or equivalent measurement of the zero carb sweetener of your choice

1/4 teaspoon xanthan gum

1/4 cup water

Makes 18 servings; Net Carbs: 3 g per serving

Preparation:

Preheat oven to 350 F.

Combine butter, flour, 1/2 cup sweetener and salt in a medium bowl until a dough just forms. Press 2/3 of the crust dough into the bottom of an 8 x 8 glass pan. Bake 7 minutes and then place it on a baking rack to cool.

Combine the blueberries, remaining sweetener, xanthan gum, and water in a small saucepan and simmer approximately 10 minutes until the mixture thickens. Stir gently to keep some blueberries intact.

With the remaining crust dough, knead the cinnamon into it well. Spread the blueberry filling evenly over the crust and pinch pieces of the topping crust over the filling. Bake 25 minutes until topping is browned.

Allow streusel to cool completely before cutting. Cut into 18 individual servings by first cutting 9 even squares and then cutting each square in half diagonally.

Peppermint Bark

Ingredients:

9 ounces sugar free chocolate chips

18 pieces of round sugar free peppermint hard candies

1 tablespoon coconut oil

1 teaspoon of peppermint extract

Makes 8 servings; Net Carbs: 2 g per 1-1/2 ounce serving

Preparation:

Line a jellyroll pan with parchment paper.

In a double boiler, melt the chocolate until completely melted with 1 Tablespoon coconut oil.

Place peppermint candy in a freezer bag and crush into small pieces. Set 2 tablespoons of this mixture aside for later.

Add the crushed candies to the melted chocolate. Immediately remove from heat and spread over the parchment paper. Try to spread it evenly into a rectangle. Quickly top the chocolate with the reserved crushed candies.

Place pan in refrigerator until chocolate is firm, about 1 hour. Cut or break into 1-1/2 ounce pieces.

Conclusion:

After reading this book, I hope that you see the benefits of the Keto diet and have the knowledge to apply it. The Keto diet doesn't need to be disrupting or limiting. It can fit easily into your current lifestyle!

Everybody will be amazed to see you eating so freely and still getting lean. Soon, you will be enjoying the attention you get.

What are you waiting for?

About the Author:

Vonnie Lynn is an educator, best-selling author, homemaker, and, (according to her husband), an all-around phenomenal cook. She lives in North-central Idaho with a husband who loves to eat, their two sons, two dogs and a cat.

Other Books by Vonnie:

The Ultimate Keto Diet Workbook for Beginners

Keto that Fits Your Lifestyle

For updates on upcoming books, click here:
VonnueLynnBooks@gmail.com

If you found my book helpful, please leave a review. Your feedback helps me help others achieve their goals and helps me improve my books!

9 781672 942393